Biomedical Imaging Demystified

A Layman's Guide to Medical Scans

Tihirou Muctarr Nicol

Other Books by The Author

1. Quantum Computing Demystified
2. Green Conspiracy
3. The Future of Space Tourism
4. Indoor Gardening
5. Soccer – My Favorite Game

Dedication

I wish to dedicate this book and extend a heartfelt "Thank You" to every purchaser and potential supporter who, at some point, responded with a "No."

I JUST MADE A SALE!

You're my new customer, and I want to express my heartfelt thanks for choosing to do business with me. Your support means the world to me, and I value your trust. In my work, which includes consulting, volunteering, and writing, I have three key goals:

1. To make a positive impact on people's lives.

2. To build strong, lasting relationships.

3. To have a blast while doing it!

When I wrote this book, my main aim was to make it incredibly useful to you. I hoped it would be so helpful that you'd happily recommend it to at least ten of your co-workers, friends, and family members. I'd love to hear from you if I've succeeded in reaching that goal.

Because of you, and all my amazing customers, I get to do what I'm passionate about – selling, writing, and teaching.

Thank you so much!

Table of Contents

Introduction to Biomedical Imaging

Hey there! Welcome to the fascinating world of biomedical imaging. If you're like me, you might be curious about how doctors and scientists use cool machines to see inside our bodies without cutting us open. Well, you're in luck because, in this chapter, we're going to dive into the basics of biomedical imaging. Don't worry; we'll keep things simple and easy to understand, even if you're in the sixth grade.

What's Biomedical Imaging, Anyway?

Imagine you have a superpower – the power to see inside your own body or someone else's, just like Superman can see through walls. Well, that's kind of what biomedical imaging is all about. It lets us peek inside the human body without using a scalpel or anything scary.

Now, why do we need to do this? Well, our bodies are like complex puzzles, and sometimes doctors need to solve these puzzles to figure out what's going on. They use biomedical imaging to see things that are hidden from the naked eye, like bones, organs, and even blood vessels. It's like having a secret superhero tool to help doctors save lives and keep us healthy.

How Does It Work?

Okay, here's the cool part. Biomedical imaging works in different ways, and we'll explore those in more detail in the chapters ahead. But for now, let's talk about the basic idea.

Most biomedical imaging techniques use special machines and energy, like X-rays, sound waves, or even radioactive stuff, to create pictures of the inside of our bodies. These pictures are like maps that doctors can use to find problems or check if everything is A-okay. Think of it as taking a snapshot of what's happening inside you.

For example, X-rays are like super-duper high-energy light beams that can pass through your body and create images of your bones. Magnetic Resonance Imaging (MRI) uses powerful magnets and radio waves to show soft things like your brain or muscles. And there are many more cool techniques we'll explore.

Why Is This Important?

Now, you might wonder why all of this matters. Well, it matters a lot! Biomedical imaging helps doctors catch diseases early, like cancer or heart problems. It guides surgeons during operations, making sure they're fixing the right stuff. And it helps researchers learn more about our bodies, which can lead to new medicines and treatments.

Imagine if you had a puzzle with missing pieces, and you didn't even know it. Biomedical imaging helps us find those missing pieces in our bodies' puzzles and put them together.

So, in this book, we'll take a closer look at the different types of biomedical imaging, like X-rays, MRIs, CT scans, and more. By the time you finish reading, you'll have a superpower of your own – the power to understand how these amazing machines work and how they help keep us healthy. Get ready to explore the incredible world of medical scans!

The Amazing History of Medical Scanning

Hey there, curious minds! Today, we're taking a time machine back through history to discover the incredible journey of medical scanning. So, buckle up, because it's going to be an exciting ride!

The Ancient Beginnings

Our story begins way, way back in ancient times. Imagine living thousands of years ago when doctors couldn't just peek inside your body like they can today. They had to rely on their keen eyes, their hands, and a good dose of guesswork.

One of the earliest forms of medical scanning was something called "percussion." No, it doesn't involve drumming; it's more like tapping your body to listen for different sounds. Doctors would tap your chest or belly to figure out what was going on inside. If it sounded hollow, it meant one thing, and if it sounded dull, it meant something else. Pretty clever, right?

X-rays: The Game Changer

Now, let's jump ahead to the late 1800s. A brilliant scientist named Wilhelm Conrad Roentgen was experimenting with some strange rays. He didn't fully understand them, but he noticed something incredible. When he aimed these rays at objects, they created mysterious images on a screen. It was like magic!

Roentgen named these rays "X-rays" because they were so mysterious. And these X-rays turned out to be a game-changer for medicine. In 1895, Roentgen took the first-ever X-ray image of his wife's hand, and the world of medical scanning was born.

Suddenly, doctors could see inside the body without cutting it open. They could diagnose broken bones, spot foreign objects, and even detect diseases like tuberculosis. X-rays quickly became the superhero tool of the medical world.

The Rise of Radiography

As X-rays gained popularity, a new field called "radiography" emerged. Radiographers were like the photographers of the medical world. They used X-ray machines to take pictures of the inside of the body, and these images were called radiographs.

In the early 1900s, radiography was all the rage. It was used to find bullets in wounded soldiers during World War I and to inspect luggage at airports. People even used to carry around their own little radiographs like souvenirs, which seems pretty strange today!

The Advent of Ultrasound

Fast forward to the 1950s. Another amazing invention came into play: ultrasound. Now, you might think of ultrasound as something that only helps expecting parents see their baby in the womb, but it's much more than that.

Ultrasound uses sound waves instead of X-rays to create images. A special device called a transducer sends out sound waves, which bounce off the body's tissues and organs, creating pictures on a screen. It's safe, painless, and super useful.

Ultrasound became a crucial tool in diagnosing various medical conditions. It allowed doctors to check the heart, liver, kidneys, and more, all without any radiation. So, it's like a gentle superhero in the world of medical scanning.

CT Scans: A 3D View

In the 1970s, a brand-new superhero joined the team: the CT scan, short for "Computed Tomography." This was a game-changer because it gave doctors a 3D view of the inside of the body.

A CT scanner is like a fancy donut-shaped machine. You lie on a table, and it slides you through the donut hole while taking lots of X-ray pictures from different angles. A computer then puts all these images together, creating a detailed 3D map of your insides.

CT scans are super helpful in finding problems like tumors, bleeding, or injuries. They allow doctors to see things from all angles, making diagnosis and treatment planning much easier.

Magnetic Resonance Imaging (MRI): A Magnet Magic Show

Now, let's talk about MRI, which stands for Magnetic Resonance Imaging. Imagine being inside a massive magnet, but don't worry; it's not as scary as it sounds.

MRI uses strong magnets and radio waves to create incredibly detailed images of your body's soft tissues like the brain, muscles, and organs. It's like a magic show where the magnet makes your body's atoms dance, and the computer turns that dance into pictures.

MRI is especially helpful when doctors need to see inside the brain or check for problems in the joints and muscles. It's like having a superhero with a cape made of magnets!

Nuclear Medicine: Radioactive Heroes

In the world of medical scanning, there are even heroes who use a bit of radioactivity for good. Nuclear medicine is all about this exciting stuff. It sounds scary, but it's not dangerous when used properly.

Here's how it works: patients are given a tiny amount of a radioactive substance that goes to a specific part of their body, like the heart or bones. A special camera then detects the radiation and creates images that show how well that part of the body is working.

Nuclear medicine helps diagnose conditions like cancer, heart disease, and bone disorders. It's like having a radioactive detective inside your body, solving mysteries for the doctors.

PET Scans: Tracking Metabolism

Speaking of superheroes, let's meet PET scans, which stands for Positron Emission Tomography. These scans are like metabolic detectives.

In a PET scan, a small amount of radioactive sugar is injected into your body. Areas with higher metabolism (where cells are super active) absorb more sugar and show up as bright spots on the scan. This helps doctors spot cancer, see how the brain is working, and track other diseases.

So, PET scans are like a map of your body's energy, helping doctors understand what's happening inside you on a cellular level.

Mammography: Superheroes for Breast Health

Ladies, this one's especially important for you. Mammography is like a superhero dedicated to breast health. It's all about early detection of breast cancer.

A mammogram is a type of X-ray that takes pictures of the breast tissue. By catching breast cancer early, doctors can save lives. It's like having a guardian angel for breast health.

Bone Scans: Checking Your Skeleton

Our bones are like the hidden heroes of our bodies, providing structure and support. But sometimes, they need a little checkup too. That's where bone scans come in.

In a bone scan, a small amount of radioactive material is injected into your bloodstream. This material travels to your bones, and a special camera takes pictures of your skeleton. It helps doctors spot bone diseases, fractures, and even infections.

So, bone scans are like the superhero sidekicks who make sure your skeleton stays strong and healthy.

Doppler Imaging: The Blood Flow Detectives

Ever wonder how doctors check blood flow in your body? They use a technique called Doppler imaging, and it's like being a blood flow detective.

Doppler imaging uses sound waves to create images of blood moving through your veins and arteries. It helps doctors spot blockages, clots, or other issues that might affect your circulation. It's like having a superhero who listens to your blood and makes sure it's flowing smoothly.

Fluoroscopy: Real-Time Radiography

Imagine if you could watch a movie of your insides in real time. That's exactly what fluoroscopy does. It's like having a live-action superhero inside you.

During a fluoroscopy procedure, a special X-ray machine continuously takes images and displays them on a screen. This is incredibly helpful during surgeries, like when a doctor needs to guide a catheter through your blood vessels or examine your digestive system.

Fluoroscopy is like the superhero film director who captures the action as it happens inside your body.

Angiography: Mapping Your Arteries

Angiography is like the cartographer of the medical world, creating detailed maps of your arteries and blood vessels. It's crucial for spotting blockages, aneurysms, or other problems that might affect your circulation.

During an angiogram, a special dye is injected into your bloodstream, making your blood vessels show up on X-ray images. It's like having a treasure map for your veins, helping doctors navigate and fix problems.

Endoscopy: A Camera Inside You

Now, let's talk about endoscopy. Imagine sending a tiny camera on a mission inside your body to explore and take pictures. That's exactly what endoscopy does.

During an endoscopy, a flexible tube with a camera at the end is inserted into your body through your mouth, nose, or other openings. It helps doctors examine your digestive tract, airways, or other internal areas. It's like having a mini explorer who goes where no one else can.

Emerging Technologies in Biomedical Imaging

As we wrap up our journey through the history of medical scanning, it's worth mentioning that technology keeps evolving. New superheroes are constantly joining the team.

For example, there are now 3D and 4D ultrasound scans that provide even more detailed images of growing babies. There are also advances in artificial intelligence (AI) that help doctors interpret medical scans more accurately and quickly.

Scientists and doctors are always working on ways to make medical scanning safer, more accessible, and more powerful. Who knows what amazing superheroes in the world of biomedical imaging we'll meet in the future?

In Conclusion

So, there you have it, the incredible history of medical scanning. From the ancient days of tapping and guessing to the modern era of high-tech machines and radioactive detectives, we've come a long way in our quest to understand and heal the human body.

Remember, these amazing technologies are like the superheroes of the medical world. They help doctors save lives, catch diseases early, and make sure we stay healthy. The next time you see a medical scan, you'll know that it's not just a picture; it's a piece of history and a symbol of human ingenuity and progress.

X-rays: Peering Inside the Body

Hey there, young explorers! Today, we're going on an exciting journey into the world of X-rays. Imagine having the power to see through walls and even through your own body – that's what X-rays are all about. So, let's dive into the magical world of X-rays and discover how they help doctors see inside us.

What Are X-rays?

First things first, what are X-rays? Well, they're a type of invisible light, sort of like the light that comes from the sun but with way higher energy. Because they have so much energy, X-rays can do something amazing – they can pass through objects that regular light can't, like your skin and muscles.

Imagine if you had a super flashlight that could shine through walls and even your own body. That's what X-rays are like for doctors. They use these special rays to look inside us and figure out what's going on.

The X-ray Machine

Now, let's talk about the magical machine that makes all this possible – the X-ray machine. It's not a giant camera or a sci-fi contraption; it's a pretty simple and safe device.

Here's how it works: You might have seen a doctor or a radiographer (that's a person who takes X-rays) holding a small, flat panel or a tube-like thing. This is the X-ray machine. When they aim it at the part of your body they want to check, it sends out a burst of X-rays.

These X-rays travel through your body and hit a special plate on the other side. The plate captures the X-rays that make it through your body, and they create a picture. It's kind of like taking a photograph, but instead of using regular light, they use X-rays.

Getting an X-ray

Now, let's talk about what it's like to get an X-ray. Have you ever seen those cool X-ray images of your bones or teeth? Maybe you've had an X-ray at the dentist to check your teeth. Well, that's just one way X-rays are used.

When you go for an X-ray, the first thing you'll do is put on a lead apron. It might look a bit like a superhero cape, but it's not for flying. This apron is there to protect the parts of your body that don't need an X-ray, like your tummy or chest.

Next, you'll be asked to stand still or lie down on a table, depending on which part of your body is being X-rayed. The radiographer will position the X-ray machine so that it's aimed at the right spot. Then, they'll step out of the room and press a button to take the X-ray picture.

Don't worry; you won't feel a thing. X-rays are painless, and you won't even notice them passing through your body. It's all over in just a few seconds, like a quick superhero mission.

Why Do We Need X-rays?

You might be wondering, "Why do we need X-rays? Can't doctors just look at us?" Well, X-rays are like a secret superpower for doctors. They help them see things that are hidden deep inside your body.

Here are a few reasons why X-rays are so important:

Finding Broken Bones: If you ever hurt yourself and think you might have broken a bone, X-rays can confirm whether it's fractured or not. This helps doctors decide on the right treatment, like putting a cast on your arm or leg.

Spotting Problems in Your Lungs: X-rays are great at showing your lungs and chest. Doctors can use them to check for things like pneumonia or if you accidentally swallowed something you shouldn't have.

Checking Your Teeth: When you visit the dentist, they might use X-rays to see what's happening inside your teeth. It helps them catch cavities early and make sure your smile stays healthy.

Finding Hidden Objects: Sometimes, kids (and even grown-ups) accidentally swallow things like coins or small toys. X-rays can help doctors locate these objects and make sure they're safely removed.

Looking at Your Joints: If you have joint pain or an injury, like a twisted ankle, X-rays can show if there's any damage to your bones or joints.

Detecting Diseases: X-rays can help doctors find diseases like lung cancer or arthritis early on when they're easier to treat.

So, you see, X-rays are like doctors' special goggles that allow them to see inside us and solve all sorts of mysteries. They help keep us healthy and make sure we get the right treatment when something's not quite right.

Are X-rays Safe?

Now, you might be wondering if X-rays are safe, and that's a great question. X-rays are generally safe when used properly. The amount of radiation you get from a single X-ray is very small, like a tiny fraction of what you'd get from natural sources, like the sun or the ground.

Doctors and radiographers take special care to make sure you get the right amount of X-rays for your specific situation. They use the lowest possible dose to get the information they need, especially when it comes to kids.

Remember that lead apron you wear during an X-ray? It's like a superhero shield that keeps the radiation away from the parts of your body that don't need to be X-rayed. So, you're well-protected.

However, it's essential to tell the doctor or radiographer if you might be pregnant because X-rays can be harmful to developing babies. They'll take extra precautions to keep both you and your little one safe.

The Future of X-rays

As we wrap up our adventure into the world of X-rays, it's worth mentioning that technology keeps advancing. Scientists and doctors are always working on making X-rays even safer and more precise.

Digital X-rays are becoming more common, which means quicker results and less exposure to radiation. Plus, there are ongoing research and developments to make X-ray machines even more efficient and to reduce radiation exposure even further.

So, the future looks bright for X-rays, and they'll continue to be an essential tool in the world of medicine, helping doctors be real-life superheroes by peering inside our bodies and keeping us healthy.

In Conclusion

There you have it, young explorers – the incredible world of X-rays. They're like invisible beams of light that doctors use to look inside us and figure out what's going on. X-rays help diagnose broken bones, spot diseases, and keep our bodies in tip-top shape.

So, the next time you see an X-ray machine, you'll know it's not just a piece of fancy equipment; it's a superhero tool that helps doctors take care of us. Keep being curious and asking questions, because that's how we learn about the amazing world of science and medicine!

MRI Magic: Unveiling Soft Tissues

Hey there, curious minds! Today, we're going to explore another incredible superhero of the medical world – the MRI machine. It's like a wizard's wand that reveals the secrets of our soft tissues, like the brain, muscles, and organs. So, get ready to dive into the mesmerizing world of MRI and discover how it works its magic.

What Does MRI Stand For?

First things first, let's crack the code. MRI stands for Magnetic Resonance Imaging. It sounds a bit like a science fiction gadget, but it's real, and it's pretty amazing.

The Power of Magnets

At the heart of an MRI machine is a powerful magnet. But don't worry; it won't pull you in like a superhero villain's evil trap. This magnet is there to create the magic.

The way it works is like this: every part of your body is made up of tiny things called atoms. These atoms are like the building blocks of life. Now, when you put your body inside the MRI machine, the magnet makes these atoms do a special dance.

Imagine the atoms spinning around like little tops. The MRI magnet makes them spin even faster and align in a certain way. Then, when the machine sends radio waves into your body, the atoms absorb the energy from these waves.

Now here's where the magic begins. When the radio waves are turned off, the atoms go back to their normal spinning. But as they do, they release energy in the form of signals. These signals are like whispers from your body's soft tissues, and the MRI machine turns them into images.

Different Soft Tissues, Different Signals

The coolest part about MRI is that it can create images of your body's soft tissues in incredible detail. Each type of soft tissue, like your brain, muscles, or organs, gives off slightly different signals, like having its own secret language.

Because of this, doctors can use MRI to get a closer look at what's happening inside your body without using any radiation, like X-rays do. It's like having a superhero microscope for your insides.

Getting an MRI

Okay, now let's talk about what it's like to get an MRI. Imagine you're going on a spaceship adventure. You'll be the astronaut, and the MRI machine will be your spaceship.

When you arrive at the MRI lab, you might need to change into a special gown. This isn't a fancy superhero costume, just something comfy without any metal, because remember, magnets are involved, and metal and magnets don't mix!

Next, you'll lie down on a table that slowly slides into the MRI machine. It might look like a giant donut or a tunnel. But don't worry; you won't get stuck. You'll have plenty of space around you, and there's a little window so you can see out.

The radiographer, who's like the captain of your spaceship, will give you some headphones or earplugs because the MRI machine can be a bit noisy. It might sound like a mix between a drumroll and a spaceship taking off. But don't let it scare you; it's just the machine doing its thing.

You'll need to lie very still, just like an astronaut during a mission. The MRI takes pictures of your body in slices, so you might need to hold your breath for a few seconds at a time. It's like taking snapshots of your body's secrets.

The whole process can take anywhere from 15 minutes to over an hour, depending on what the doctor needs to see. But don't worry; you won't be alone. The radiographer will keep an eye on you from their control room and make sure you're comfortable.

Once your MRI adventure is over, you can hop off the spaceship table and go back to your regular clothes. The doctor will look at the images and use them to figure out what's happening inside your body.

Why Do We Need MRI?

Now that you know how MRI works, you might be wondering why we need it. Well, MRI is like a superhero detective that helps doctors solve mysteries and catch problems early. Here are some of the super important things MRI can do:

Check Your Brain: MRI is terrific at creating detailed images of your brain. It helps doctors spot issues like tumors, strokes, or injuries.

Look at Muscles and Joints: If you hurt a muscle or a joint, MRI can show if there's any damage. It's like having a magnifying glass for your body's moving parts.

Explore Your Organs: MRI can peek inside your organs, like your heart, liver, or kidneys. It's helpful for diagnosing diseases or checking how well they're working.

Detect Problems in Your Spine: If you have back pain or spine issues, MRI can capture images of your spine's soft tissues and help doctors figure out the cause.

Examine Your Blood Vessels: MRI can also be used to look at your blood vessels and find blockages or problems with your circulation.

So, you see, MRI is a superhero tool that helps doctors keep you healthy. It's like having a magical camera that takes pictures of your body's secrets and helps find and fix any trouble.

Are MRIs Safe?

You might be wondering if MRIs are safe, and the answer is yes, they are very safe. In fact, MRI doesn't use any radiation like X-rays do, so you don't have to worry about radiation exposure.

However, there are a few things to keep in mind:

Metal and Magnets Don't Mix: Remember, the MRI machine has a powerful magnet, so it's super important to tell the doctor or radiographer if you have any metal in your body. Things like braces, piercings, or even medical implants could be affected.

Claustrophobia: Some people feel a bit claustrophobic inside the MRI machine because it's like being in a tunnel. But don't worry; you can always ask for a cloth to cover your eyes or even some relaxing music to make you feel more comfortable.

Loud Noises: As I mentioned earlier, the MRI machine can be noisy, but it's harmless. The headphones or earplugs they give you will help.

Pregnancy: If you're pregnant or might be pregnant, it's essential to let the doctor know because they'll take extra precautions to keep you and your baby safe.

The Future of MRI

As we wrap up our journey into the world of MRI, it's exciting to know that technology keeps advancing. Scientists and engineers are working hard to make MRI even better and more comfortable for patients.

One exciting development is the use of stronger magnets, which can create even more detailed images faster. This means shorter MRI scans and more comfort for patients, especially kids.

Also, researchers are exploring new techniques to make MRI images even clearer and easier for doctors to interpret. Plus, they're working on making MRI machines more accessible and affordable, so more people can benefit from this amazing technology.

In Conclusion

There you have it, young explorers – the incredible world of MRI. It's like having a magic wand that reveals the secrets of your soft tissues. MRI helps doctors diagnose diseases, check your brain, muscles, organs, and so much more, all without any radiation.

So, the next time you hear about someone having an MRI, you'll know that they're using a superhero tool to keep them healthy and discover the mysteries hidden inside their bodies. Keep being curious, and who knows, maybe one day you'll become a real-life superhero in the world of medicine!

CT Scans: Navigating the 3D World

Hey there, fellow adventurers! Today, we're strapping on our exploration boots and diving headfirst into the fascinating world of CT scans. CT stands for Computed Tomography, and it's like having a magical 3D map of the inside of your body. So, get ready for an exciting journey as we learn how CT scans work and why they're so important.

The CT Scanner: A 3D Mapmaker

Alright, imagine you're exploring a massive cave, and you want to see every twist and turn in its dark depths. How would you do that? With a flashlight, of course! Well, in the world of medicine, the CT scanner is like that super-duper flashlight.

CT scanners are like big donut-shaped machines, and they're your ticket to the 3D world inside your body. When you lie on the CT table and slide into the scanner, it's like embarking on a fantastic voyage. You're about to create a detailed 3D map of your insides.

X-Rays and Computers: The Dynamic Duo

Now, let's talk about how CT scanners work their magic. You see, they use X-rays, just like the ones we talked about when exploring X-rays. But here's the twist – CT scanners take lots and lots of X-ray pictures from different angles.

It's like having a team of photographers snapping shots of you from all sides while you strike different poses. These pictures are like puzzle pieces, and the CT scanner's computer puts them together to form a 3D image.

The computer is the real hero here. It's super fast and can process all those X-ray images in a flash. It takes the information from each picture and creates a detailed 3D map that shows everything – bones, organs, blood vessels, and more.

Why Do We Need CT Scans?

Great question! CT scans are incredibly useful, and they're like treasure maps for doctors. Here are some reasons why we need them:

Finding Hidden Problems: If you have a mysterious pain or an illness that's hard to diagnose, CT scans can help doctors get to the bottom of it. They can spot things like tumors, infections, or injuries hiding inside your body.

Planning Surgery: When a doctor needs to perform surgery, they want to know exactly what they're getting into. CT scans give them a sneak peek of your insides, so they can plan the operation with precision.

Checking for Diseases: CT scans are excellent at finding diseases like cancer, heart disease, or lung problems. Early detection is often the key to successful treatment, and CT scans can help with that.

Monitoring Health: If you have a chronic condition like diabetes or heart disease, CT scans can help doctors keep tabs on how things are progressing. It's like having a health checkup for your insides.

Assessing Injuries: If you're in an accident or have a sports injury, CT scans can quickly show if there are any broken bones, internal bleeding, or other issues that need immediate attention.

Getting a CT Scan

Okay, let's imagine you're going for a CT scan. What's it like? Well, it's a bit like taking a ride through a space tunnel, but don't worry, it's not as scary as it sounds.

First, you'll change into a comfy hospital gown, and the radiographer (that's the person who operates the CT scanner) will explain what's going to happen. They might ask you to remove any jewelry or metal objects because these can interfere with the scan.

You'll lie down on the CT table, which looks like a narrow bed, and get comfy. The radiographer will make sure you're in the right position, and then they'll move the table into the donut-shaped scanner.

The CT machine is pretty quiet compared to an MRI, but it can still make some buzzing and whirring noises. You might be given headphones or earplugs to block out the noise and make the experience more comfortable.

Once you're all set up, the CT scanner will start taking pictures. You might need to hold your breath for a few seconds at a time so that the images come out as clear as possible. It's like trying to take a steady picture with your camera while standing very still.

The whole process usually takes just a few minutes, and then you're free to go! You can get back to your regular activities right away because there's no recovery time needed.

Are CT Scans Safe?

Absolutely, CT scans are considered safe when used by trained professionals. However, because they use X-rays, which are a form of radiation, doctors try to use the lowest amount of radiation necessary to get the job done.

For most people, the small amount of radiation from a CT scan is not a big concern. But if you've had multiple CT scans or are very sensitive to radiation, your doctor will take extra precautions.

It's always a good idea to let your doctor know if you're pregnant because radiation exposure can be harmful to developing babies. In such cases, doctors will consider other imaging options, like ultrasound or MRI, if possible.

The Future of CT Scans

Now, let's take a quick peek into the future of CT scans. Technology is always advancing, and CT scanners are getting better and better.

One exciting development is the use of lower-dose CT scans. Scientists are finding ways to reduce the amount of radiation used during the scan while still getting high-quality images. This is great news because it makes CT scans even safer.

Researchers are also working on making CT scans faster and more efficient, so you spend less time inside the scanner. That means quicker results and a more comfortable experience for patients, especially kids who might find staying still a bit challenging.

In Conclusion

There you have it, fellow adventurers – the incredible world of CT scans! They're like 3D maps that help doctors explore your insides and solve medical mysteries.

The next time you hear someone talk about getting a CT scan, you'll know that they're using a fantastic tool to keep their health in check. Keep being curious, and who knows, maybe one day you'll become a medical explorer using CT scans to help others stay healthy and happy!

Ultrasound: Sound Waves in Medicine

Hey there, inquisitive minds! Today, we're going on a fantastic voyage into the world of ultrasound. Ultrasound is like a superhero with super-hearing, using sound waves to help doctors see inside your body. So, let's embark on this exciting journey and discover how ultrasound works its magic!

What Is Ultrasound?

First things first, let's break it down. Ultrasound is like sending sound waves into your body and listening to the echoes they bounce back. It's kind of like how a bat uses echolocation to find its way in the dark.

The device that sends and receives these sound waves is called an "ultrasound machine." It's a bit like a magic wand that helps doctors see what's happening inside you without any radiation or cutting you open.

How Does Ultrasound Work?

Now, you might be wondering how this whole ultrasound thing works. It's pretty cool, actually. The ultrasound machine has a small device called a "transducer," which looks a bit like a microphone or a small wand. It's the superhero sidekick in this story.

When your doctor or a trained technician places the transducer on your skin, they apply a special gel to help the sound waves travel smoothly. Then, the transducer sends out tiny sound waves that are too high-pitched for your ears to hear – kind of like dog whistles.

These sound waves travel through your skin and bounce off the organs and tissues inside your body. When they bounce back to the transducer, it listens carefully and turns the echoes into pictures on a screen.

It's a bit like how you can tell if a room is empty or full just by shouting and listening to the echoes. Ultrasound does the same thing, but it's super precise and quick.

Why Do We Need Ultrasound?

You might be wondering why we need ultrasound when we already have X-rays and CT scans. Well, ultrasound has its own set of superpowers that make it essential in the world of medicine. Here's why:

No Radiation: Unlike X-rays and CT scans, ultrasound doesn't use any radiation. This makes it super safe, especially for pregnant women and kids. You can have an ultrasound as often as needed without worrying about harmful radiation exposure.

Real-Time Action: Ultrasound is like a live-action superhero. It provides real-time images, which means doctors can see what's happening inside your body right at that moment. This is incredibly useful during surgeries or when monitoring a developing baby during pregnancy.

Soft Tissues and Organs: While X-rays and CT scans are great at showing bones, ultrasound excels at revealing soft tissues and organs. It's like having a backstage pass to explore your heart, liver, kidneys, and even an unborn baby.

Painless and Non-Invasive: Getting an ultrasound is a breeze. It's painless, and there are no needles or cutting involved. You just lie back and let the ultrasound machine do its thing.

Versatile: Ultrasound is like a Swiss Army knife of medical imaging. It can be used for a wide range of purposes, from checking your baby's growth during pregnancy to diagnosing conditions like gallstones or kidney problems.

Getting an Ultrasound

Alright, let's say you need an ultrasound. What's it like? Well, it's pretty straightforward, and there's nothing to worry about.

Preparing for the Ultrasound: Depending on the type of ultrasound you're getting, you might need to follow specific instructions before the appointment. For example, if you're having an abdominal ultrasound, you might need to avoid eating for a few hours before the test. Your healthcare provider will let you know if any preparations are needed.

The Ultrasound Room: When you arrive at the ultrasound clinic, you'll be greeted by a friendly technician. They'll lead you to the ultrasound room, which usually has a comfy examination bed and the ultrasound machine.

Getting Ready: To get the best pictures, you'll need to expose the part of your body that's being examined. If it's your abdomen, you might need to lift or remove your shirt. If it's your pelvis, you might be asked to change into a gown.

The Ultrasound Procedure: The technician will apply a special gel to your skin, which helps the sound waves travel better. Then, they'll use the transducer to gently glide over the area. You might feel a bit of pressure, but it's usually painless and quite comfortable.

Watching the Screen: The technician will keep an eye on the screen as they move the transducer. You can also watch the screen if you're curious! You might see the images, which look a bit like black and white pictures. The technician will capture the important images they need for the doctor.

Wrapping Up: Once the images are captured, the technician will clean off the gel from your skin, and you can get dressed if you have to change into a gown. They'll let you know if you're all set or if the doctor needs more images.

Getting the Results: Your doctor will review the ultrasound images and discuss the findings with you. They might use the ultrasound to confirm a diagnosis, monitor the progress of a pregnancy, or check on the health of your organs.

Are Ultrasounds Safe?

Yes, ultrasounds are incredibly safe. There's no radiation involved, so you don't have to worry about any harmful effects. Doctors have been using ultrasound for many years, and it's a trusted and well-established medical tool.

Ultrasounds are even used during pregnancy to monitor the growth and health of the developing baby. They're so safe that pregnant women often have multiple ultrasounds during their pregnancy to ensure everything is on track.

The Future of Ultrasound

As we wrap up our journey into the world of ultrasound, it's exciting to know that technology keeps advancing. Researchers and scientists are always working on making ultrasound even more powerful and versatile.

One exciting development is the use of 3D and 4D ultrasound. These techniques provide incredibly detailed images and even allow doctors to see moving images, like a baby's movements in the womb. It's like watching a live-action movie of your insides!

Additionally, portable ultrasound devices are becoming more accessible. These smaller machines are like pocket-sized superheroes that can be used in remote areas or during emergencies to quickly assess and diagnose medical conditions.

In Conclusion

There you have it, curious minds – the fantastic world of ultrasound! It's like sending sound waves on a mission to explore your body and create detailed images that help doctors keep you healthy.

The next time you hear someone talking about getting an ultrasound, you'll know that they're using a powerful tool that's safe, painless, and incredibly useful in the world of medicine. Keep being curious, because who knows, you might become a real-life superhero in the field of healthcare one day.

Nuclear Medicine: Radioactive Insights

Hey there, curious explorers! Today, we're going on a fascinating adventure into the world of nuclear medicine. It's like having a tiny superhero, called a "tracer," injected into your body to help doctors see what's going on inside. So, buckle up as we dive into the world of nuclear medicine and uncover how it works its radioactive magic!

What Is Nuclear Medicine?

First things first, let's demystify nuclear medicine. It's not about nuclear bombs or anything scary like that. Nuclear medicine is a branch of medical imaging that uses tiny amounts of radioactive substances to look inside your body.

These radioactive substances are often called "radiotracers" or "radiopharmaceuticals." They're like special messengers that carry a little bit of radiation with them. When they're injected into your body, they go on a mission to specific areas, and their radiation helps create images that reveal what's happening inside you.

How Does Nuclear Medicine Work?

Now, you might be wondering how this radioactive magic happens. It all starts with the radiotracer. Imagine it as a secret agent with a tiny radioactive backpack.

When you get a nuclear medicine scan, the radiotracer is either injected into your bloodstream, swallowed as a pill, or inhaled as a gas, depending on what your doctor needs to check. Once it's inside your body, the radiotracer starts its journey.

The radiotracer gives off small particles called gamma rays. These gamma rays are a bit like invisible beams of light, and they're detected by a special camera called a "gamma camera" or a "SPECT scanner." It's like having a superhero camera that can see things your regular camera can't.

As the radiotracer moves through your body, the gamma camera captures the gamma rays it emits. The camera then turns these rays into images that doctors can see on a computer screen. These images show the distribution of the radiotracer and help doctors understand what's happening inside your body.

Why Do We Need Nuclear Medicine?

Nuclear medicine might sound a bit out of this world, but it has some super important uses in the world of medicine. Here are a few reasons why it's a valuable tool:

Detecting Diseases: Nuclear medicine is like a disease detective. It can help doctors spot diseases in their early stages when they're easier to treat. For example, it's used to find cancer, heart problems, and bone disorders.

Evaluating Organ Function: Sometimes, it's not just about seeing what something looks like; it's about understanding how it works. Nuclear medicine can assess the function of organs like the heart, liver, and kidneys to make sure they're doing their jobs correctly.

Guiding Treatment: Nuclear medicine can also be used to plan and monitor treatments. For instance, it helps doctors figure out the right dosage for radiation therapy or check if a treatment is working.

Studying How the Body Works: It's like having a backstage pass to watch your body's inner workings. Researchers use nuclear medicine to study various bodily processes, from blood flow to bone growth.

Checking for Infections: Nuclear medicine can help doctors find infections or areas of inflammation in the body. It's like a superhero tool for diagnosing hidden trouble.

Getting a Nuclear Medicine Scan

Alright, let's say you need a nuclear medicine scan. What's it like? Don't worry; it's not as intimidating as it sounds.

Preparation: Before your scan, your healthcare provider will explain what's going to happen and answer any questions you have. Depending on the type of scan, you might need to follow specific instructions. For example, if you're having a bone scan, you might need to drink extra water before the procedure.

The Radiotracer: Next comes the radiotracer, our tiny radioactive superhero. It's either injected into your vein, given as a pill, or inhaled, depending on the type of scan and what your doctor needs to check.

The Wait: Once the radiotracer is inside your body, you might need to wait for a little while. This gives the radiotracer time to reach the area of interest.

The Scan: Now, it's time for the scan itself. You'll be asked to lie on a comfortable examination table. The gamma camera or SPECT scanner will be positioned over the area being examined. It might move around or take images from different angles. It's like having a superhero camera that captures the action from all sides.

Hold Still: During the scan, it's super important to stay still. Just like a superhero needs a steady hand to capture the perfect shot, the gamma camera needs you to be still so that the images come out clear and accurate.

The End: Once the scan is complete, you're free to go! There's usually no recovery time needed, and you can get back to your regular activities.

Are Nuclear Medicine Scans Safe?

Yes, nuclear medicine scans are considered safe when performed by trained professionals. The amount of radiation from a radiotracer is typically very small and poses minimal risk to your health. Doctors carefully choose the type and amount of radiotracer based on your specific needs.

That said, if you're pregnant or think you might be pregnant, it's essential to let your healthcare provider know. In such cases, they'll take extra precautions or consider alternative imaging methods to ensure the safety of both you and your baby.

The Future of Nuclear Medicine

As we wrap up our adventure into the world of nuclear medicine, it's exciting to know that technology keeps advancing. Scientists and researchers are continually working on improving the techniques and safety of nuclear medicine scans.

One exciting development is the use of more targeted radiotracers. These are like having super-smart superheroes that go directly to the problem area, reducing radiation exposure to the rest of the body.

Additionally, advancements in imaging technology are making nuclear medicine scans even more precise and efficient. This means quicker and more accurate diagnoses, which is fantastic news for patients.

In Conclusion

There you have it, intrepid explorers – the captivating world of nuclear medicine! It's like having a secret agent, the radiotracer, giving off tiny bits of radiation to help doctors see what's happening inside you.

The next time you hear someone talk about nuclear medicine, you'll know that they're using a powerful tool to diagnose, treat, and monitor various medical conditions. Keep being curious, because who knows, maybe one day you'll be part of the team pushing the boundaries of nuclear medicine to help people live healthier lives!

PET Scans: Tracking Metabolism

Hey there, fellow adventurers! Today, we're setting off on an exciting journey into the world of PET scans. PET stands for Positron Emission Tomography, and it's like having a high-tech camera that tracks the secret lives of your body's cells. So, fasten your seatbelts as we dive into the world of PET scans and uncover how they work their metabolic magic!

What Is a PET Scan?

First things first, let's demystify PET scans. They're not about your furry friends; they're about your body's inner workings. PET scans are a special type of imaging that helps doctors see how your cells are working.

Imagine if you could put on a pair of magic glasses and see the energy activity inside your body's cells. Well, that's kind of what a PET scan does. It allows doctors to watch your cells in action and understand how they're using energy.

How Does a PET Scan Work?

Okay, now let's get into the nitty-gritty of how PET scans actually work. At the heart of a PET scan is a special substance called a "radiotracer." Think of it as a tiny explorer that carries a bit of radiation with it.

The radiotracer is made up of molecules that are similar to those your body uses for energy. It's like having a spy that looks just like the locals. When you get a PET scan, the radiotracer is usually injected into your vein.

Once it's inside your body, the radiotracer starts to act like a detective. It goes to areas where your cells are super active and using a lot of energy. These could be places like your heart, brain, or tumors.

Now, here's the cool part. When the radiotracer gets to these active areas, it releases tiny particles called "positrons." Positrons are like the clues that the detective leaves behind. They don't stick around for long; they quickly find their "partner in crime," which is an electron, and they both vanish.

But before they disappear, the positron and electron collide, creating a burst of energy. This burst of energy is what PET scans detect. It's like a flash of light in the darkness, and it tells the PET scanner where the radiotracer has been and where your cells are using energy.

The PET scanner has detectors all around it, and they pick up these flashes of energy. The computer then turns these signals into images that show the areas with high metabolic activity.

Why Do We Need PET Scans?

You might be wondering why we need PET scans when we already have X-rays and other types of imaging. Well, PET scans have their own unique superpowers that make them invaluable in the world of medicine. Here's why they're so important:

Metabolic Insight: PET scans are like metabolic detectives. They show how your cells are using energy, which can help doctors spot diseases and conditions early. For example, they're excellent at detecting cancer, brain disorders, and heart diseases.

Tailored Treatment: When you're battling a disease, like cancer, doctors need to know if the treatment is working. PET scans can track changes in metabolic activity, helping doctors adjust your treatment plan if needed.

Brain Function: PET scans can peer into the brain and reveal how different areas are functioning. This is super helpful for diagnosing brain disorders like Alzheimer's disease and epilepsy.

Cardiac Clarity: They're fantastic at looking at the heart's metabolism, helping doctors understand heart conditions and plan treatments like bypass surgery.

Research Tool: PET scans are also used in medical research to study various conditions and how different treatments affect the body's metabolism.

Getting a PET Scan

Alright, let's say you need a PET scan. What's it like? Don't worry; it's not as daunting as it might seem.

Preparation: Before your PET scan, your healthcare provider will give you specific instructions. This could include fasting for a few hours before the scan, depending on what's being examined. It's essential to follow these instructions to ensure the best results.

Radiotracer Injection: When you arrive at the imaging center, you'll be given the radiotracer. It's typically injected into a vein in your arm. You might feel a slight pinch, but it's usually not painful.

Waiting Period: After the injection, you'll need to wait for a while. This gives the radiotracer time to spread throughout your body and accumulate in areas of high metabolic activity.

The PET Scan: Once it's time for the scan, you'll lie down on a comfy examination table. The table moves into the PET scanner, which looks like a big donut. You'll need to stay very still during the scan, just like when taking a photo.

During the Scan: The PET scanner will start capturing images as it moves around you. It might take a little while, but it's painless, and you can even listen to music or relax during the procedure.

Post-Scan: Once the scan is complete, you're good to go! There's usually no recovery time, and you can resume your regular activities.

Are PET Scans Safe?

Absolutely, PET scans are considered safe when performed by trained professionals. The amount of radiation from the radiotracer is relatively low and won't harm your body. However, it's essential to discuss the risks and benefits with your doctor, especially if you're pregnant or breastfeeding.

The Future of PET Scans

As we wrap up our adventure into the world of PET scans, it's exciting to know that technology keeps advancing. Scientists and researchers are continuously working to make PET scans even more precise and accessible.

One exciting development is the use of new radiotracers. These are like having more specific detectives that can uncover even smaller details about metabolic activity. This can lead to earlier disease detection and more tailored treatments.

Additionally, advancements in imaging technology are making PET scans faster and more comfortable for patients. This means shorter scan times and less time spent inside the scanner, which is great news for those who might find it challenging to stay still for long periods.

In Conclusion

There you have it, adventurous minds – the captivating world of PET scans! It's like having a metabolic detective that tracks how your cells use energy to reveal important health insights.

The next time you hear someone talk about having a PET scan, you'll know that they're using a powerful tool to monitor their health, detect diseases early, and tailor treatments to their unique needs. Keep being curious, because who knows, maybe one day you'll be part of the team advancing the field of PET scans to help people live healthier lives!

Mammography: Screening for Breast Health

Hey there, awesome readers! Today, we're diving into the world of mammography, a superhero in the world of medical imaging. Mammography is like having a special X-ray machine designed just for your breasts. It's all about keeping your breast health in check, and we're here to unravel the secrets of how it works and why it's essential.

What Is Mammography?

Let's start with the basics. Mammography is a kind of X-ray imaging that focuses on your breasts. It's like taking a sneak peek inside your chest to see what's going on in there. But why do we need it, you ask? Well, it's like having a superpower to spot potential issues in your breast tissue, especially when it comes to breast cancer.

How Does Mammography Work?

Now, let's get into the nitty-gritty of how mammography actually works. It's not as complicated as it might sound!

The Mammogram Machine: First, you'll meet the mammogram machine. It's like a big camera that takes X-ray pictures of your breasts. There are two plates on the machine—one on top and one on the bottom.

Compression: Here's the part that might sound a little uncomfortable, but it's super important. To get a clear picture, your breast needs to be pressed gently between the two plates. Don't worry; it's quick, and the pressure doesn't last long.

X-ray Beams: The mammogram machine then sends a tiny burst of X-ray beams through your breast. These beams are like invisible rays of light that pass through the tissue.

Images Captured: On the other side of your breast, there's a detector that captures the X-ray images. These images show what's happening inside your breast tissue. Think of it as a secret snapshot of your breast's inner world.

Repeat for the Other Breast: The same process is repeated for your other breast. This way, doctors can compare both sides to make sure everything looks okay.

The whole process usually takes just a few minutes for each breast, and you're in and out of the clinic pretty quickly.

Why Do We Need Mammograms?

Great question! Mammograms play a crucial role in keeping your breast health in check. Here's why they're so important:

Early Detection: Mammograms are like early warning alarms for breast cancer. They can detect lumps or changes in your breast tissue before you or your doctor can feel them. Catching breast cancer early often means better treatment options and a higher chance of a full recovery.

Monitoring Changes: If you've had breast cancer before or have a family history of it, regular mammograms help doctors keep a close eye on any changes in your breast tissue. It's like having a superhero guardian watching over your health.

Guiding Treatment: If you're diagnosed with breast cancer, mammograms help doctors plan the best course of treatment. They can see the size and location of the tumor, which helps in deciding on surgery, radiation, or chemotherapy.

Peace of Mind: For many people, getting a clean bill of health after a mammogram is like a huge sigh of relief. It provides peace of mind and reassurance that everything is okay.

Getting a Mammogram

Alright, let's say you're due for a mammogram. What's it like? It's totally normal to have questions, but the process is pretty straightforward:

Scheduling: Your doctor or a screening center will schedule your mammogram. They'll choose a time when your breasts are less likely to be tender, which is usually during the first half of your menstrual cycle if you're premenopausal.

Preparing: On the day of your mammogram, try to wear a two-piece outfit. This makes it easier to undress from the waist up when it's time for the scan. Avoid using deodorants, lotions, or powders on your chest area because they can interfere with the images.

Arriving at the Clinic: When you arrive, you'll be asked a few questions about your medical history, so it's a good idea to have that information handy.

The Mammogram: You'll be taken to the mammogram room, where a friendly mammography technologist will guide you through the process. They'll position your breast on the machine and gently compress it between the two plates to get clear images.

Hold Still: While the X-ray pictures are being taken, it's essential to hold very still. This helps ensure that the images come out sharp and clear.

Repeat for the Other Breast: The process is then repeated for your other breast. The technologist will make sure both sides are checked thoroughly.

Waiting for Results: After the mammogram, you might need to wait a bit for the results. Don't worry if you're a bit anxious during this time; it's entirely normal.

Are Mammograms Painful?

You might have heard that mammograms can be a bit uncomfortable because of the compression. While it's true that the pressure can feel strange, it's usually not painful, and it lasts only for a few seconds. Remember, this moment of mild discomfort can help ensure your breast health and early detection of any potential issues.

Mammograms and Radiation Exposure

You might be concerned about radiation exposure during a mammogram. It's a valid concern, but the amount of radiation used in mammography is very low and considered safe. The benefits of early breast cancer detection far outweigh the small radiation dose you receive during the exam.

The Future of Mammography

As we wrap up our journey into the world of mammography, it's exciting to know that technology keeps advancing. Researchers and scientists are continually working to make mammograms even better and more comfortable for patients.

One exciting development is the use of 3D mammography, also known as digital breast tomosynthesis. This technology provides more detailed images and reduces the chances of false positives or callbacks for additional testing.

Additionally, researchers are exploring ways to improve the comfort of mammograms, making the experience even less intimidating for patients.

In Conclusion

There you have it, amazing readers — the incredible world of mammography! It's like having a superhero X-ray machine focused on keeping your breast health in check and catching potential issues early.

The next time you hear someone talk about getting a mammogram, you'll know that they're taking a proactive step to protect their health and potentially save lives. Keep being curious, because staying informed about your health is a superpower in itself!

Bone Scans: Examining the Skeletal System

Hey there, fellow adventurers! Today, we're going on a journey deep into the world of bone scans. These amazing scans are like having a special map to explore your skeletal system. Whether it's to find hidden fractures or check the health of your bones, bone scans are here to help, and we're about to uncover how they work and why they matter.

What Is a Bone Scan?

Let's start with the basics. A bone scan is a kind of medical imaging that's all about your bones. It's like using a secret camera that can see what's happening inside your skeleton. But why do we need it? Well, it's like having a superhero tool to spot any bone problems, like fractures or bone diseases.

How Does a Bone Scan Work?

Now, let's dive into the nitty-gritty of how bone scans actually work. It's not as complicated as it might seem!

The Radiotracer: At the heart of a bone scan is a special substance called a "radiotracer." Think of it as a tiny explorer with a flashlight. This radiotracer is usually a small amount of radioactive material that's mixed with a special liquid.

Getting the Radiotracer: You'll receive the radiotracer through an injection into one of your veins. It's like giving the explorer a backpack filled with a tiny flashlight.

Waiting for a Bit: Once the radiotracer is inside your body, you might need to wait for a little while. This gives it time to spread throughout your skeleton, just like our explorer finding their way through a dark cave.

The Scan Begins: Now, it's time for the bone scan itself. You'll lie down on an examination table, and a special camera is placed above you. This camera can detect the tiny bit of radiation that the radiotracer gives off.

Capturing the Images: The camera slowly moves over your body, taking pictures of your bones. It's like snapping photos of the explorer's journey through the cave. The camera doesn't touch you, and you won't feel anything during this part.

Different Views: Sometimes, the camera might take pictures from different angles to get a better look at specific areas. It's like using a flashlight to explore every nook and cranny of the cave.

Creating the Images: All the pictures taken by the camera are sent to a computer. The computer processes them and turns them into detailed images of your bones. It's like developing photos from the explorer's journey.

These images show your doctor how your bones are doing, whether they're healthy, or if there are any issues to address.

Why Do We Need Bone Scans?

You might be wondering why we need bone scans when we already have X-rays and other types of imaging. Well, bone scans have their own unique superpowers that make them essential in the world of medicine. Here's why they matter:

Detecting Hidden Fractures: Bone scans are like detectives for hidden fractures. Sometimes, regular X-rays can't spot them, but bone scans can, helping doctors figure out the cause of unexplained pain.

Checking for Bone Diseases: Conditions like osteoporosis and bone infections can weaken your bones without obvious symptoms. Bone scans can reveal these issues before they become major problems.

Cancer Detection: Bone scans are excellent at spotting areas of the bone that might be affected by cancer. They help doctors determine the extent of cancer's spread, which guides treatment decisions.

Monitoring Healing: After a bone injury or surgery, bone scans can track how well your bones are healing. It's like having a progress report on your body's repair work.

Planning Treatment: When it comes to bone diseases or cancer that has spread to the bones, bone scans provide vital information for treatment planning. They help doctors decide on the best course of action.

Getting a Bone Scan

Alright, let's say you need a bone scan. What's it like? Don't worry; it's not as intimidating as it might sound.

Preparation: Before your bone scan, your healthcare provider will give you specific instructions. These might include avoiding certain medications or fasting for a few hours before the scan.

Releasing the Radiotracer: When you arrive at the imaging center, you'll receive the radiotracer through an injection into one of your veins. It's like giving the explorer their backpack and flashlight.

The Wait: After the injection, you might need to wait for a little while. This gives the radiotracer time to spread throughout your bones.

The Bone Scan: Now, it's time for the bone scan itself. You'll lie down on an examination table, and the camera is positioned above you. The camera will move slowly over your body, taking pictures of your bones.

Holding Still: During the scan, it's essential to stay very still. This helps ensure that the images come out clear and accurate. The scan is painless, and you won't feel anything.

Post-Scan: Once the scan is complete, you're good to go! There's usually no recovery time needed, and you can resume your regular activities.

Are Bone Scans Safe?

Yes, bone scans are considered safe when performed by trained professionals. The amount of radiation you receive from the radiotracer is relatively low and poses minimal risk to your health. Doctors carefully choose the type and amount of radiotracer based on your specific needs.

The Future of Bone Scans

As we wrap up our adventure into the world of bone scans, it's exciting to know that technology keeps advancing. Researchers and scientists are continually working to make bone scans even more precise and efficient.

One exciting development is the use of more targeted radiotracers. These are like having super-smart explorers who can pinpoint specific bone issues, reducing the amount of radiation exposure to the rest of your body.

Additionally, advancements in imaging technology are making bone scans faster and more comfortable for patients. This means shorter scan times and less time spent at the imaging center.

In Conclusion

There you have it, adventurous minds – the intriguing world of bone scans. It's like having a special map to explore your skeletal system and uncover any hidden secrets your bones might be hiding.

The next time you hear someone talk about getting a bone scan, you'll know that they're using a powerful tool to keep their bones healthy and address any issues that might arise. Keep being curious, because staying informed about your health is a superpower in itself.

Doppler Imaging: Blood Flow in Focus

Hello, curious minds! Today, we're setting off on an exciting adventure into the world of Doppler imaging. It's like having a magic wand that lets doctors see how blood flows through your body. Whether it's checking your heart, your baby in the womb, or finding blocked arteries, Doppler imaging is here to help, and we're going to uncover how it works and why it's so important.

What Is Doppler Imaging?

Let's start with the basics. Doppler imaging is a type of medical ultrasound that's all about blood flow. It's like having a superhero stethoscope that can actually show the movement of blood inside your veins and arteries. But why is that so cool, you ask? Well, it's like having a secret window to understand how your heart and blood vessels are doing.

How Does Doppler Imaging Work?

Now, let's dive into the nitty-gritty of how Doppler imaging actually works. It's not as complicated as it might sound!

The Doppler Effect: To understand Doppler imaging, we need to know about the "Doppler Effect." It's like when a car with a siren approaches you and then moves away. The sound changes pitch as it comes closer (higher pitch) and moves away (lower pitch). The same happens with waves, like sound or ultrasound.

Sending and Receiving Waves: In Doppler imaging, a device sends out high-frequency sound waves. These waves are like tiny messengers sent into your body. They bounce off things like blood cells and return to the device.

Listening to the Echo: When the waves bounce back, the device listens to them. If the blood cells are moving toward the device (like a car approaching you), the waves get compressed, and they sound higher-pitched. If the blood cells are moving away from the device (like a car moving away from you), the waves get stretched, and they sound lower-pitched.

Creating the Image: The device uses these changes in pitch to create images. It's like drawing a map of how fast and in which direction the blood is flowing. These images help doctors understand what's happening inside your body.

Why Do We Need Doppler Imaging?

Great question! Doppler imaging plays a crucial role in the world of medicine. Here's why it's so important:

Checking Your Heart: Doppler imaging can help doctors look at your heart and blood vessels. It's like having a special mirror to see how well your heart is pumping blood and if there are any problems with the blood flow.

Pregnancy Magic: During pregnancy, Doppler imaging is like a peek inside the womb. It helps doctors make sure the baby is getting enough oxygen and nutrients through the placenta.

Vascular Insights: When it comes to your blood vessels, Doppler imaging is like a superhero detective. It can spot blocked or narrowed arteries, which might lead to conditions like stroke or heart disease.

Blood Clot Alert: It's also used to detect blood clots in your veins. This is crucial because if a blood clot breaks free, it can travel to your lungs or brain, causing serious problems.

Monitoring Health: Doppler imaging helps doctors monitor chronic conditions like diabetes, where blood flow problems can occur over time. It's like a health check-up for your blood vessels.

Getting a Doppler Imaging Test

Alright, let's say you need a Doppler imaging test. What's it like? Don't worry; it's not as intimidating as it might seem.

Preparation: Depending on what part of your body is being examined, your healthcare provider might ask you to wear comfortable clothing and avoid using lotions or oils on your skin. They'll give you specific instructions, so be sure to follow them.

The Test: You'll be asked to lie down on an examination table, and a warm gel is applied to the area being examined. This gel helps the sound waves travel better. It's usually quite soothing, like a cozy blanket for your skin.

The Device: The technician will use a handheld device called a "transducer." This device emits the sound waves and also listens to the echoes bouncing back. It's gently moved over the area being examined.

Listening to the Waves: As the technician moves the transducer, you might hear the sound of the waves. This is the Doppler effect in action! The technician is listening to the echoes to create the images.

Holding Still: During the test, it's important to stay as still as possible. This helps get clear images. You might be asked to change positions or take deep breaths at times, but it's usually painless and comfortable.

Post-Test: Once the images are captured, the test is complete, and you're good to go! There's usually no recovery time needed, and you can resume your regular activities.

Is Doppler Imaging Safe?

Absolutely, Doppler imaging is considered safe when performed by trained professionals. It uses sound waves instead of radiation, so there's no exposure to harmful radiation. It's one of the safest imaging methods out there.

The Future of Doppler Imaging

As we wrap up our adventure into the world of Doppler imaging, it's exciting to know that technology keeps advancing. Researchers and scientists are continually working to make Doppler imaging even more precise and versatile.

One exciting development is the use of 3D and 4D Doppler imaging. This means not only can doctors see the blood flow but also how it changes over time. It's like having a real-time movie of your body's inner workings.

Additionally, portable Doppler devices are becoming more accessible. These handheld gadgets are like pocket-sized superheroes that can be used in remote areas or during emergencies to quickly assess blood flow and diagnose problems.

In Conclusion

There you have it, intrepid explorers – the fascinating world of Doppler imaging. It's like having a magic wand that reveals the mysteries of blood flow in your body.

The next time you hear someone talk about getting a Doppler imaging test, you'll know that they're using a powerful tool to check their heart, monitor pregnancy, or detect problems in their blood vessels. Keep being curious, because who knows, you might be the one pushing the boundaries of Doppler imaging to help people live healthier lives.

Fluoroscopy: Real-Time Radiography

Hello, my curious friends! Today, we're diving into the world of fluoroscopy, a fascinating medical technique that's like having a magic window into your body. It's all about real-time radiography, and whether it's guiding surgeons during procedures or diagnosing digestive issues, fluoroscopy is here to dazzle us. So, let's uncover how it works, why it's essential, and why it's such an exciting part of medical imaging.

What is Fluoroscopy?

Let's start with the basics. Fluoroscopy is a kind of medical imaging that gives doctors a live, moving look at the inside of your body. It's like watching a movie of your body's inner workings in real-time. But why is that so amazing, you ask? Well, it helps doctors see how your organs function and perform various procedures with precision.

How Does Fluoroscopy Work?

Now, let's get into the nitty-gritty of how fluoroscopy actually works. It's not as complicated as it might sound!

The Fluoroscope Machine: At the heart of fluoroscopy is a special machine called a "fluoroscope." It's like a superhero camera that can capture moving images inside your body.

X-Rays at Play: Just like in regular X-rays, fluoroscopy uses X-rays too, but with a twist. Instead of taking one static image, it sends continuous X-ray beams through your body. It's like having a spotlight shining inside you.

Fluorescent Screen: Behind your body, there's a special screen that can glow when hit by X-rays. It's like a canvas that lights up when the X-rays pass through your body.

Real-Time Images: As the X-rays pass through you, they create real-time images on the fluorescent screen. These images show what's happening inside your body at that very moment.

Detecting Movement: Here's the coolest part: the fluoroscope is super sensitive to movement. So, if you're having a fluoroscopy of your stomach while drinking a contrast agent (a special liquid that shows up on X-rays), the machine can capture how your stomach moves as you swallow.

Watching Live: The images created by the fluoroscope are shown on a monitor in the examination room. This way, both you and your doctor can watch what's happening inside your body in real-time.

Why Do We Need Fluoroscopy?

Great question! Fluoroscopy plays a vital role in the world of medicine. Here's why it's so important:

Guiding Procedures: Doctors often use fluoroscopy to guide them during procedures like placing a stent in a blocked blood vessel or inserting a catheter into your bladder. It's like having a GPS for your insides, ensuring precision and safety.

Digestive Diagnostics: For digestive problems, fluoroscopy is a superhero tool. It helps doctors see how your stomach, esophagus, and intestines work. It's like having a live-action movie of your digestive system.

Orthopedic Insights: Orthopedic surgeons use fluoroscopy to see how bones and joints move during surgery. It's like having an X-ray camera to guide them in fixing broken bones or performing joint replacements.

Cardiac Clarity: Cardiologists use fluoroscopy to watch the heart in action. It's like having a front-row seat to see how your heart's valves and chambers are doing.

Pulmonary Precision: Pulmonologists can use fluoroscopy to visualize your lungs and airways in real time. It helps them diagnose and treat lung conditions more effectively.

Getting a Fluoroscopy Exam

Alright, let's say you need a fluoroscopy exam. What's it like? Don't worry; it's not as intimidating as it might seem.

Preparation: Depending on what part of your body needs to be examined, your healthcare provider will give you specific instructions. For digestive exams, you might need to fast for a few hours before the test.

The Exam Room: You'll be taken to the fluoroscopy room, where there's a fluoroscope machine and a monitor.

The Contrast Agent: If your exam involves the digestive system, you might be asked to drink a contrast agent. This liquid helps highlight your organs on the X-ray images.

Getting Positioned: You'll need to be positioned in a way that allows the fluoroscope to capture the best images. It's like finding the perfect angle for a photograph.

Real-Time Viewing: During the exam, the fluoroscope machine will start taking real-time X-ray images. If you're having a procedure, like getting a stent, the doctor will watch the images on the monitor to guide them.

Watching and Waiting: If you're awake during the procedure, you can watch the monitor to see what's happening inside your body. It's like having a front-row seat to your own show!

Post-Exam: Once the exam is done, you'll receive any necessary follow-up instructions, like whether you can eat or drink. In most cases, there's no recovery time needed, and you can go about your day.

Is Fluoroscopy Safe?

Yes, fluoroscopy is considered safe when performed by trained professionals. However, it does involve exposure to X-rays, so it's essential to use the lowest possible dose needed for accurate images. Doctors are careful to balance the benefits of the exam with the small amount of radiation used.

The Future of Fluoroscopy

As we wrap up our adventure into the world of fluoroscopy, it's exciting to know that technology keeps advancing. Researchers and scientists are continually working to make fluoroscopy even safer and more efficient.

One exciting development is the use of digital fluoroscopy. This technology provides clearer and more detailed images while using lower doses of radiation. It's like having a sharper and safer window into your body.

Additionally, portable fluoroscopy machines are becoming more common. These compact devices can be easily moved around the hospital, making it more convenient for patients who need real-time imaging during procedures.

In Conclusion

There you have it, adventurous minds – the incredible world of fluoroscopy! It's like having a magic window that lets doctors watch your body in action, helping them diagnose, treat, and guide procedures with precision.

The next time you hear someone talk about getting a fluoroscopy exam, you'll know that they're using a powerful tool to gain real-time insights into their health. Keep being curious, because who knows, maybe one day you'll be part of the team pushing the boundaries of fluoroscopy to help people live healthier lives!

Angiography: Mapping Your Arteries

Hey there, curious minds! Today, we're embarking on a fascinating journey into the world of angiography. It's like having a treasure map for your arteries, helping doctors discover and understand the highways of your blood flow. Whether it's diagnosing blockages or guiding life-saving procedures, angiography is here to amaze us. So, let's dive into how it works, why it's crucial, and why it's such an incredible part of medical imaging.

What is Angiography?

Let's start with the basics. Angiography is a special kind of medical imaging that's all about your blood vessels. It's like having a secret camera that captures detailed pictures of your arteries and veins. But why is that so important, you ask? Well, it helps doctors see if there are any problems with blood flow, like blockages or narrow spots.

How Does Angiography Work?

Now, let's uncover the magic of how angiography actually works. It's not as complicated as it might sound!

The Contrast Agent: At the heart of angiography is a special dye called a "contrast agent." Think of it as a tiny explorer that makes your blood vessels stand out on X-ray images. This dye is usually injected into a blood vessel, often in your groin or arm.

X-Ray Machine: Just like in regular X-rays, angiography uses X-ray machines, but they are specially designed to capture images of blood vessels. It's like having a super-powered camera that can see inside your body.

The Journey of the Dye: Once the contrast agent is injected, it travels through your bloodstream, flowing along with your blood. It's like marking the path for our explorer so we can see where they've been.

X-Ray Pictures: As the dye moves through your blood vessels, the X-ray machine takes pictures. These pictures show the contrast agent highlighting your arteries and veins. It's like taking snapshots of your blood vessels in action.

Real-Time Viewing: The best part is that these X-ray images are shown on a monitor in the examination room. This means both you and your doctor can watch in real-time as the dye flows through your blood vessels.

Why Do We Need Angiography?

Great question! Angiography plays a vital role in the world of medicine. Here's why it's so important:

Detecting Blockages: Angiography is like a detective for blocked or narrowed blood vessels. It helps doctors find the places where blood flow might be restricted, which can lead to heart attacks, strokes, or other serious issues.

Guiding Procedures: It's like a GPS for surgeons and interventional radiologists. They use angiography to guide them during procedures like placing stents (tiny tubes) in blocked arteries or treating aneurysms (weakened blood vessel walls).

Diagnosing Diseases: Angiography can help diagnose diseases related to blood vessels, like atherosclerosis or vascular malformations. It's like having a magnifying glass to see the details.

Monitoring Progress: For people who've had procedures or surgeries to improve blood flow, angiography helps doctors check how well things are working. It's like a progress report on your vascular health.

Getting an Angiography

Alright, let's say you need an angiography. What's it like? Don't worry; it's not as intimidating as it might seem.

Preparation: Before your angiography, your healthcare provider will give you specific instructions. These might include fasting for a few hours before the test or letting them know about any allergies you have.

The Procedure Room: You'll be taken to the angiography suite, which is like a special room equipped with an X-ray machine and monitors.

The Contrast Agent: The contrast agent is usually injected into a blood vessel in your groin or arm. It's like our tiny explorer getting ready to map out your blood vessels.

X-Ray Pictures: As the contrast agent flows through your blood vessels, the X-ray machine captures images. It's like taking a photo album of your arteries and veins.

Real-Time Viewing: If you're awake during the procedure, you can watch the monitor to see your blood vessels light up as the contrast agent moves through them. It's like having a front-row seat to the show.

Holding Still: It's important to stay as still as possible during the procedure to get clear images. The entire process is usually painless, and you might only feel a mild sensation when the contrast agent is injected.

Post-Procedure: Once the angiography is done, you might need to rest for a bit to make sure you're feeling okay. Your healthcare team will monitor you and provide any necessary post-procedure care.

Is Angiography Safe?

Yes, angiography is considered safe when performed by trained professionals. The contrast agent contains a small amount of radiation, but the benefits of accurate diagnosis and treatment guidance far outweigh the small radiation dose.

The Future of Angiography

As we wrap up our journey into the world of angiography, it's exciting to know that technology keeps advancing. Researchers and scientists are continually working to make angiography even safer and more precise.

One exciting development is the use of less invasive techniques. Some angiography procedures can now be done through tiny incisions or even from inside your blood vessels, reducing the need for more extensive surgeries.

Additionally, 3D angiography is becoming more common. This technology creates detailed three-dimensional images of blood vessels, providing even more information for doctors and improving the accuracy of procedures.

In Conclusion

There you have it, adventurous spirits — the mesmerizing world of angiography! It's like having a treasure map for your arteries, helping doctors navigate the intricate highways of your blood flow.

The next time you hear someone talk about getting an angiography, you'll know that they're using a powerful tool to diagnose and treat blood vessel issues and ensure that blood flows smoothly throughout their body. Keep being curious, because who knows, you might be the one pushing the boundaries of angiography to help people live healthier lives!

Endoscopy: A Camera Inside You

Hey there, curious explorers! Today, we're embarking on an incredible journey into the world of endoscopy. It's like having a tiny camera that can travel inside your body, exploring places that doctors need to see up close. Whether it's diagnosing stomach issues, checking your colon, or even performing surgery without big incisions, endoscopy is here to amaze us. So, let's uncover how it works, why it's so important, and why it's such a fantastic part of medical technology.

What is Endoscopy?

Let's start with the basics. Endoscopy is a remarkable medical procedure that uses a special instrument called an endoscope. This instrument is like a super-smart camera attached to a long, thin tube. It helps doctors examine your insides without making big cuts or surgeries. Instead, they simply guide the endoscope through natural openings in your body. How cool is that?

How Does Endoscopy Work?

Now, let's dive into the magic of how endoscopy actually works. It's not as complicated as it might sound!

The Endoscope: At the heart of endoscopy is the endoscope itself. It's like having a mini-submarine with a camera on board. The endoscope can be flexible or rigid, depending on where it needs to go in your body.

The Light and Camera: The endoscope has a powerful light and a tiny camera at the tip. This camera is like having a curious explorer's eye that can capture detailed images of what it sees.

Natural Openings: To explore your insides, doctors use natural openings in your body, like your mouth, throat, or the other end. They gently insert the endoscope through these openings, so there's no need for major surgeries.

Real-Time Viewing: The camera inside the endoscope sends live images to a monitor in the examination room. This way, both you and your doctor can watch what's happening inside your body in real-time.

Guiding Tools: Sometimes, endoscopes have special tools attached, like tiny forceps or scissors. These tools are used for procedures like removing polyps or taking tissue samples.

Why Do We Need Endoscopy?

Fantastic question! Endoscopy plays a crucial role in the world of medicine. Here's why it's so important:

Diagnosis: Endoscopy is like a detective's magnifying glass. It helps doctors see the inside of your body and find out what's causing problems. For example, it can diagnose conditions like ulcers, acid reflux, or even certain cancers.

Treatment: Sometimes, endoscopy is not just for looking but for doing. Doctors can use it to treat various issues, like removing growths, stopping bleeding, or placing small devices like stents.

Preventive Care: It's like an early warning system. Endoscopy can help find and remove precancerous growths, preventing more serious conditions from developing.

Less Invasive Surgery: For some surgeries, endoscopy can be used instead of traditional open surgeries. This means smaller incisions, less pain, and a faster recovery.

Exploring Deep: Endoscopy can reach places in your body that would be difficult or impossible to see otherwise, like deep in your digestive system or your airways.

Types of Endoscopy

Endoscopy isn't one-size-fits-all; there are different types for different parts of the body:

Upper Endoscopy (Esophagogastroduodenoscopy or EGD): It's like a voyage down the food pipe. The endoscope is guided through your mouth and throat to examine your esophagus, stomach, and the first part of your small intestine.

Colonoscopy: This one explores your large intestine, or colon. The endoscope is gently inserted through your back end to check for issues like polyps or signs of colorectal cancer.

Bronchoscopy: Think of it as a trip to the lungs. The endoscope goes through your mouth or nose and down into your airways to diagnose and treat lung problems.

Gastroscopy: Similar to upper endoscopy, it focuses on your stomach and the upper part of your digestive system.

Cystoscopy: This endoscope is like a diving bell for your urinary system. It goes through your urethra to check your bladder and urinary tract.

Laparoscopy: While not exactly an endoscopy, it's worth mentioning. It's like having tiny cameras and instruments inserted through small incisions in your abdomen for surgeries like removing the appendix.

Getting an Endoscopy

Alright, let's say you need an endoscopy. What's it like? Don't worry; it's not as intimidating as it might seem.

Preparation: Before your endoscopy, your healthcare provider will give you specific instructions. This might include fasting for several hours before the procedure or adjusting medications.

Anesthesia: Depending on the type of endoscopy and your comfort level, you might receive sedation or anesthesia. It's like taking a little nap during the procedure.

Insertion: The endoscope is gently inserted through a natural opening in your body. The healthcare team ensures you're comfortable and relaxed.

Real-Time Viewing: If you're awake during the procedure, you can watch the monitor to see your insides up close. It's like having an educational adventure through your own body.

Procedure or Biopsy: If needed, the doctor can perform procedures or take small tissue samples during the endoscopy. It's like having a handy toolbox inside your body.

Recovery: After the endoscopy, you'll be taken to a recovery area to wake up fully. You might feel a bit drowsy, but it wears off quickly. If you had anesthesia, you'll need someone to drive you home.

Is Endoscopy Safe?

Absolutely! Endoscopy is considered very safe when performed by trained professionals. It's a minimally invasive procedure that reduces the risks and complications associated with traditional open surgeries. Any potential risks are usually outweighed by the benefits of accurate diagnosis and treatment.

The Future of Endoscopy

As we wrap up our adventure into the world of endoscopy, it's exciting to know that technology keeps advancing. Researchers and scientists are continually working to make endoscopy even more precise and comfortable for patients.

One exciting development is the use of miniaturized instruments and robotics. These tiny tools can be guided by doctors through the endoscope, allowing for more complex and delicate procedures.

Additionally, advancements in imaging technology are making endoscope cameras even more powerful, providing clearer and more detailed images of your insides.

In Conclusion

There you have it, intrepid explorers – the remarkable world of endoscopy! It's like having a tiny camera that can travel inside your body, helping doctors diagnose, treat, and explore without major surgeries.

The next time you hear someone talk about getting an endoscopy, you'll know that they're using a fantastic tool to get a close-up look at their insides and ensure their health. Keep being curious, because who knows, maybe you'll be part of the team pushing the boundaries of endoscopy to help people live healthier lives!

Emerging Technologies in Biomedical Imaging

Hello, inquisitive minds! Today, we're venturing into the exciting world of emerging technologies in biomedical imaging. It's like discovering the latest gadgets and tools that doctors use to see inside our bodies. These new advancements are revolutionizing the way we diagnose, treat, and understand our health. So, let's embark on this journey to explore the future of medical imaging and how it's making our lives healthier and better.

What is Biomedical Imaging, Anyway?

Before we dive into the shiny new stuff, let's quickly review what biomedical imaging is all about. Biomedical imaging is like having a magic window that lets doctors see inside our bodies without actually opening us up. It's a bit like superheroes using their X-ray vision but in real life.

Now, let's get to the exciting part – the emerging technologies that are changing the game.

Artificial Intelligence (AI) and Machine Learning:

Imagine having a super-smart assistant who can look at medical images and instantly spot even the tiniest of problems. Well, that's what AI and machine learning are bringing to the world of biomedical imaging.

How It Works:

AI algorithms are trained on massive amounts of medical image data. They learn to recognize patterns and abnormalities. When they see a new image, they can quickly analyze it and flag anything that looks unusual.

Why It's Cool:

This technology can help doctors diagnose diseases like cancer much earlier, leading to better outcomes. It also reduces the chances of human error, making healthcare more precise.

3D Printing:

Picture this – your doctor has a perfect replica of your heart or a bone in their hands, all thanks to 3D printing. This technology is like a magic printer that can create physical models of body parts.

How It Works:

Doctors use CT or MRI scans to create detailed 3D models of the body. Then, a 3D printer transforms these models into physical objects, which can be used for surgical planning and education.

Why It's Cool:

Surgeons can practice tricky procedures on these 3D-printed models before doing the real thing on a patient. It's like having a rehearsal before the big show, making surgeries safer and more successful.

Nanotechnology:

Think super, super tiny! Nanotechnology involves working with incredibly small materials, even smaller than a grain of sand. In biomedical imaging, nanotechnology is like having a swarm of tiny detectives inside your body.

How It Works:

Tiny particles or "nanoprobes" are designed to target specific areas in the body, like tumors. They can carry dyes or chemicals that show up on imaging scans. When they reach their target, they light up, revealing what's happening at a cellular level.

Why It's Cool:

Nanotechnology can help doctors detect diseases at their earliest stages when they're easier to treat. It's like having a sneak peek into the microscopic world of your body.

Augmented Reality (AR):

Ever played a video game with virtual objects superimposed on the real world? Well, AR is like that but in medicine. It can take medical imaging to a whole new level.

How It Works:

Surgeons wear special glasses or use devices that overlay medical images onto the patient's body during surgery. This helps them see vital information without taking their eyes off the patient.

Why It's Cool:

AR can guide surgeons with pinpoint accuracy during procedures. It's like having a GPS for surgery, reducing the risk of errors and making surgeries faster.

Wireless Capsule Endoscopy:

Remember endoscopy, where we explored the inside of the body with a tiny camera? Well, imagine if that camera were a small, swallowable capsule. That's exactly what wireless capsule endoscopy is all about!

How It Works:

You swallow a small capsule that contains a tiny camera. As it travels through your digestive system, it captures images and sends them wirelessly to a receiver worn on your body. Doctors can then review the images later.

Why It's Cool:

It's a game-changer for diagnosing digestive issues. No more uncomfortable tubes or sedation for endoscopy – just a simple swallow!

Magnetic Resonance Imaging (MRI) at Ultra-High Fields:

Regular MRI scans are already pretty amazing, but imagine having an MRI that's super-powered! Ultra-high field MRI is like having a high-resolution camera for your insides.

How It Works:

These powerful MRI machines use much stronger magnets than standard ones. This allows for incredibly detailed images of your body's structures and functions.

Why It's Cool:

It's like having a sharper and more detailed look at what's going on inside you. Doctors can spot problems earlier and with greater precision.

Photoacoustic Imaging:

This is like having a superhero with a keen sense of hearing and sight. Photoacoustic imaging combines laser light and ultrasound to create detailed images of tissues and blood vessels.

How It Works:

A laser sends pulses of light into the body. When this light hits tissue, it creates tiny vibrations. Ultrasound sensors then pick up these vibrations and turn them into images.

Why It's Cool:

It's especially useful for imaging blood vessels and tumors. It's like having a high-tech radar system for your body's hidden mysteries.

Quantum Dots:

These are tiny, glow-in-the-dark particles that can be used to tag specific cells or tissues in the body.

How It Works:

Quantum dots are engineered to emit different colors of light. By attaching them to specific molecules, they can highlight particular cells or structures during imaging.

Why It's Cool:

This technology allows doctors to track cells in real time. It's like having tiny beacons inside your body, guiding doctors to where they need to be.

Why These Advances Matter

You might be wondering why all these fancy technologies are such a big deal. Well, here's why:

Early Detection: Many of these technologies help doctors find diseases at their earliest stages when they're easier to treat. It's like catching a small problem before it becomes a big one.

Precision Medicine: With detailed imaging and data, doctors can tailor treatments to each individual's unique needs. It's like having a personalized roadmap to better health.

Reduced Risk: Advanced imaging techniques can make surgeries and procedures safer by providing doctors with more information and better tools. It's like having a safety net during medical procedures.

Less Invasive: Many of these technologies are less invasive, meaning they reduce the need for surgeries and lengthy hospital stays. It's like having medical care that's gentler on your body.

In Conclusion

There you have it, curious explorers. A glimpse into the incredible world of emerging technologies in biomedical imaging. It's like having a sneak peek into the future of healthcare, where doctors can see, diagnose, and treat with greater precision than ever before.

The next time you hear about these amazing technologies, you'll know that they're not just sci-fi fantasies – they're real tools that are changing the way we understand and care for our bodies. Keep being curious, because who knows, maybe you'll be the one to push the boundaries of biomedical imaging to make the world a healthier place.

About The Author

Welcome to my world! I'm Tihirou Nicol, a retired civil engineer turned entrepreneur, with a passion for soccer, writing, gardening, and a vision to make a difference in the world.

Background and Education

Originally hailing from the vibrant city of Freetown, Sierra Leone, I attended the esteemed Methodist Boys High School, where I nurtured my love for soccer. My academic journey then led me to Fourah Bay College, the second oldest university in Africa, where I pursued a Bachelor's Degree in Civil Engineering. Driven by a thirst for knowledge and expertise, I further honed my skills, earning a Master's Degree in Civil Engineering.

A Journey of Transformation

Throughout my professional career, I specialized in the challenging realm of road construction. However, as life unfolded, I embarked on a transformational journey that eventually led me to a diverse range of ventures.

From Civil Engineering to Business

After a fulfilling career with Kier Construction in the United Kingdom, I made a bold decision to venture into the world of entrepreneurship. I embraced the challenges and opportunities that lay ahead, starting my property business in London before relocating to the United States to continue my entrepreneurial pursuits.

Embracing My Passion: Soccer

Beyond the world of business, my heart belongs to soccer. From my school days, I actively played the beautiful game until an injury altered my path. Nevertheless, my passion for soccer endured, and I am now the proud owner of a soccer shopping outlet, where I contribute to the sport that has shaped my life.

A Commitment to Community

Even as my entrepreneurial endeavors keep me busy, I find solace in giving back to the community. I actively support my local soccer team, East End Lions, as well as the legendary Liverpool Football Club, both of which hold a special place in my heart.

A Writer and Gardener

In addition to my other passions, I am also an avid writer and gardener. I have authored several books, spanning both academic and fiction genres, many of which are available on Amazon. My writing allows me to explore new worlds and ideas, sharing my thoughts and experiences with a wider audience. When I'm not writing or tending to my business ventures, you can often find me in the garden, nurturing plants and finding solace in nature.

Seeking Honest Feedback

I value your thoughts and opinions. If you've had the chance to read any of my books, I kindly ask for an honest review or feedback. To show my appreciation, I'm offering a limited-time opportunity to receive a free copy of my upcoming book when it's published. Simply leave an honest, unbiased review on the site or bookstore where you purchased this book, and you'll be among the first to receive my next work. Your reviews helped me grow as a writer and storyteller, and I'm grateful for your support.

Motivated by Dreams

In my journey, I have drawn inspiration from visionaries like Sir Richard Branson. My aspiration is to create a positive impact on people's lives, helping them achieve their dreams and desires.

Philosophy and Approach

Hard work, perseverance, and creativity are the cornerstones of my approach to life and business. I am always seeking innovative ways to overcome challenges and find better solutions to achieve success.

A Future Full of Ambitions

Looking ahead, I envision a future with multiple shopping outlets across Sierra Leone, London, and Maryland, USA, contributing to the growth of economies and societies while continuing to indulge my passion for soccer, writing, and gardening.

Thank you for joining me on this journey of exploration and growth. Together, let's build a world where dreams come true, and where the love for soccer, the written word, and the beauty of nature unite people from all walks of life.